This Notebook Belongs To:

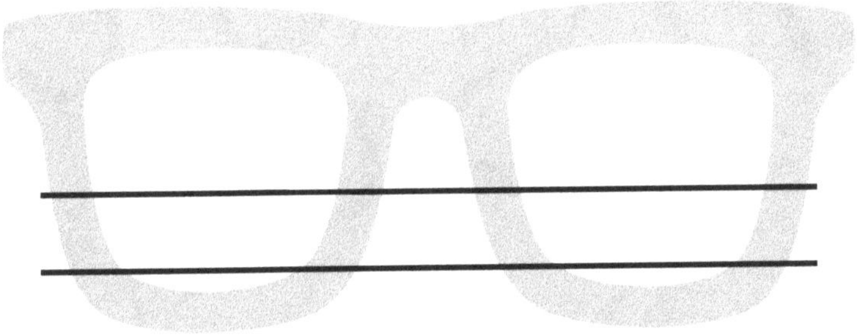

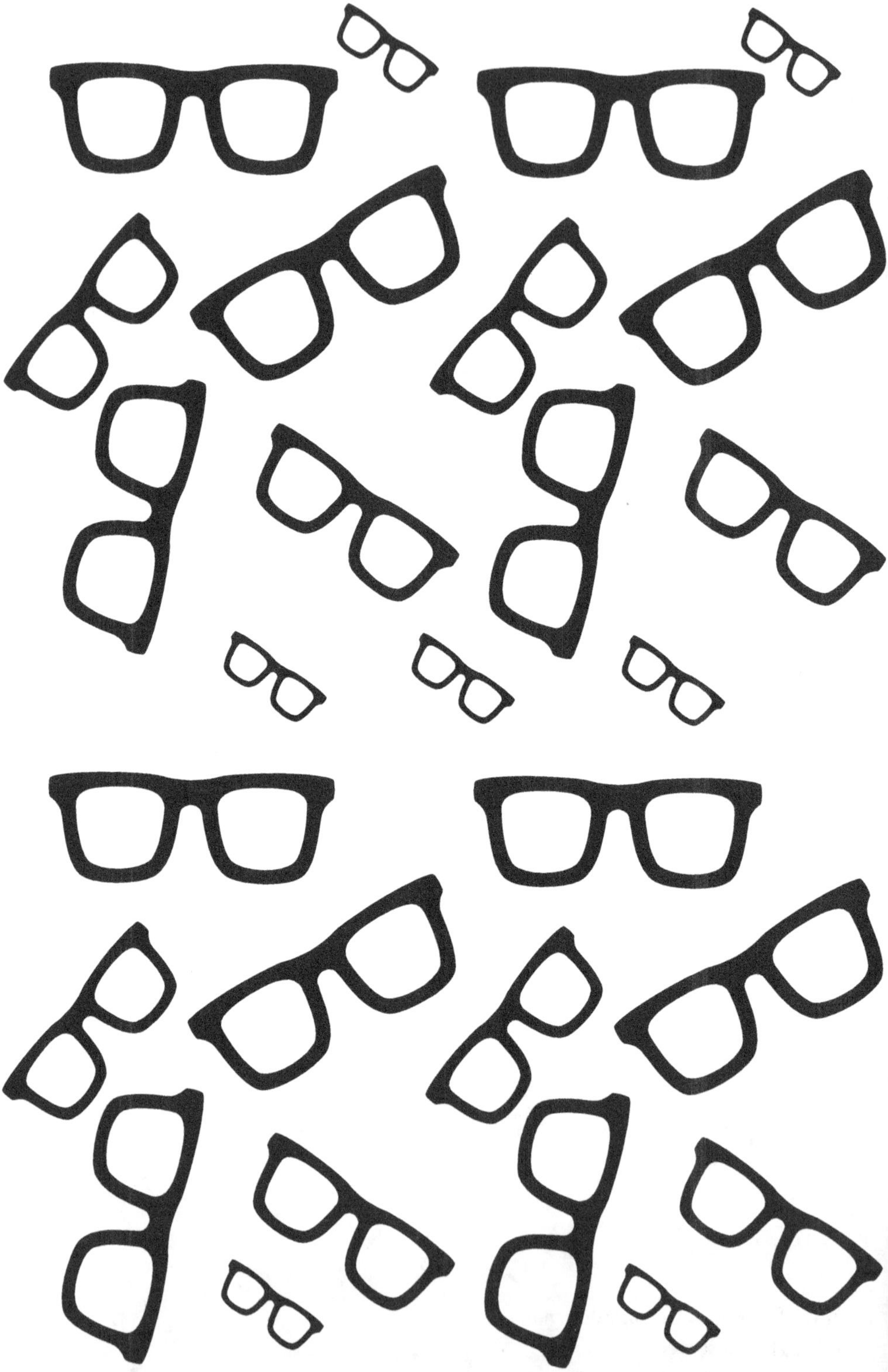

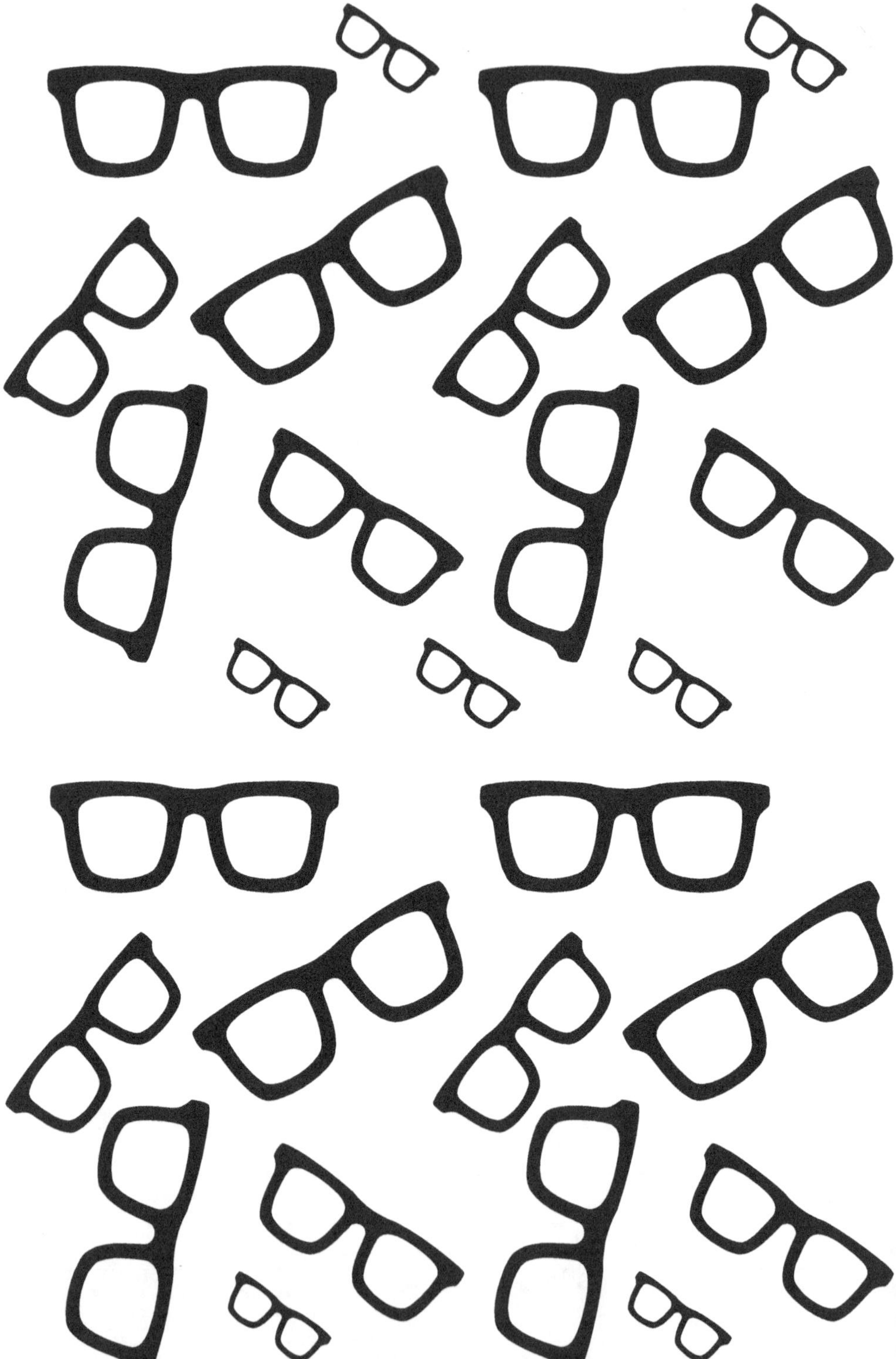

www.ingramcontent.com/pod-product-compliance
Lightning Source LLC
Chambersburg PA
CBHW070652220526
45466CB00001B/402
* 9 7 8 1 6 7 6 5 1 4 7 2 5 *